THE PEPTIDE THERAPY BIBLE

**Cutting-Edge Treatments Explained +
Innovations In Peptide Therapy & More**

DR. KYREN STEVEN

Copyright © 2024 By Dr. Kyren Steven

All Rights Reserved...

Table of Contents

Introductory 6

CHAPTER ONE 9

  Importance In Biological Systems 9

  Classification Based On Structure And Function 13

CHAPTER TWO 20

  Examples Of Therapeutic Peptide Families 20

  How Peptides Interact With Biological Targets 26

CHAPTER THREE 32

  Signaling Pathways And Cellular Responses 32

  Methods For Designing Therapeutic Peptides 38

CHAPTER FOUR 46

  Techniques In Peptide Synthesis 46

  Challenges And Innovations In Peptide Delivery 54

CHAPTER FIVE 63

  Routes Of Administration And Formulation Strategies 63

Applications Of Peptide Therapy For Alzheimer's, Parkinson's, Etc. 72

CHAPTER SIX 81

Neuroprotective Peptides And Their Mechanisms 81

Peptide Hormones In Diabetes Management 90

CHAPTER SEVEN 98

Growth Hormone Therapies And Beyond .. 98

Peptide Vaccines And Immune Modulation 107

CHAPTER EIGHT 116

Applications In Autoimmune Diseases 116

Peptides In Targeted Cancer Therapies 123

CHAPTER NINE 132

Tumor Targeting And Anti-Angiogenic Peptides 132

Peptide Treatments For Heart Conditions 140

CHAPTER TEN 147

Vasodilators And Cardiac Peptides 147

Peptides In Dermatology And Wound Care 156

CHAPTER ELEVEN 163
   Cosmeceuticals And Regenerative Medicine 163
   Issues In Peptide Stability And Bioavailability 172
   Conclusion 184
THE END..187

Introductory

Peptides are molecules composed of amino acids linked together by peptide bonds. They are smaller than proteins, typically consisting of fewer than 50 amino acids, whereas proteins are generally larger and more complex. Peptides play crucial roles in biological processes such as signaling, enzyme function, and as structural components within cells and tissues.

Key characteristics of peptides include:

• **Amino Acid Composition:** Peptides are made up of amino acids that are linked together in a specific sequence dictated by the genetic code.

• **Peptide Bonds:** These bonds form between the carboxyl group of one amino acid and the amino group of another, resulting in a peptide bond (-CO-NH-).

- **Types and Functions:** Peptides can have diverse functions based on their sequence and structure. They can act as hormones (e.g., insulin), neurotransmitters (e.g., endorphins), antibiotics (e.g., bacteriocins), or signaling molecules (e.g., neuropeptides).

- **Size Range:** Peptides can vary greatly in size, from just a few amino acids (oligopeptides) to larger chains nearing the size of small proteins. The distinction between peptides and proteins is somewhat arbitrary but often revolves around size and complexity.

- **Synthesis and Role:** Peptides are synthesized in cells through the process of translation, where messenger RNA (mRNA) directs the assembly of amino acids into specific peptide sequences. They play critical roles in maintaining biological functions and are essential components of life.

Overall, peptides are fundamental molecules in biochemistry and biology, with applications ranging from pharmaceuticals to biochemical research and beyond.

CHAPTER ONE
Importance In Biological Systems

Peptides play crucial roles in biological systems due to their diverse functions and widespread presence across various organisms. Here are some key reasons why peptides are important in biological systems:

- **Hormonal Regulation:** Peptides serve as hormones that regulate physiological processes. Examples include insulin, which regulates glucose metabolism, and oxytocin, which influences social bonding and reproductive behaviors.

- **Neurotransmission:** Many neurotransmitters in the nervous system are peptides. These molecules transmit signals between neurons, influencing mood, cognition, pain perception, and other neurological functions. Examples include endorphins, which modulate pain perception and mood, and substance P, which is involved in pain sensation.

- **Enzymatic Activity:** Peptides can act as enzymes, catalyzing biochemical reactions within cells. For instance, proteases are peptides that break down proteins, facilitating digestion and other metabolic processes.

- **Structural Support:** Peptides contribute to the structural integrity of cells and tissues. Collagen and elastin, for example, are peptides that provide strength and elasticity to connective tissues like skin, tendons, and cartilage.

- **Immune Response:** Peptides play a role in the immune system, where they function as antimicrobial agents (e.g., defensins) and antigen-presenting molecules that initiate immune responses against pathogens.

- **Cell Signaling:** Peptides act as signaling molecules that regulate cellular processes such as growth, differentiation, and apoptosis (programmed cell death). For instance, growth factors like epidermal growth factor (EGF) and transforming growth factor-beta (TGF-β) are peptide signals that control cell proliferation and tissue repair.

- **Pharmaceutical Applications:** Peptides have significant therapeutic potential. Peptide-based drugs are designed to target specific receptors or enzymes involved in disease processes, offering precise and effective treatments with fewer side effects compared to traditional drugs.

- **Research Tools:** Peptides are essential tools in biochemical and pharmaceutical research. They are used to study protein structure and function, investigate biological pathways, and develop new therapeutic strategies.

Overall, peptides are integral components of biological systems, contributing to a wide range of physiological processes essential for life, health, and adaptation to environmental challenges. Their versatility and specificity make them invaluable in both natural biology and biomedical applications.

Classification Based On Structure And Function

Peptides can be classified based on their structure and function, which reflects their diverse roles in biological systems. Here's a classification based on these criteria:

<u>Classification Based on Structure:</u>

Linear Peptides:

- Linear peptides are composed of a straightforward linear sequence of amino acids connected by peptide bonds. They can vary greatly in length and are typically synthesized using solid-phase peptide synthesis (SPPS).

Cyclic Peptides:

• Cyclic peptides form a closed ring structure due to covalent bonds between amino acids within the peptide chain. This cyclization often enhances stability and can influence their biological activity. Examples include cyclosporine and some antibiotics.

Disulfide-Bridged Peptides:

• Peptides that contain one or more disulfide bridges (covalent bonds formed between cysteine residues) are called disulfide-bridged peptides. These bridges provide structural stability and can affect their bioactivity. Examples include oxytocin and insulin.

Peptidomimetics:

• Peptidomimetics are molecules designed to mimic the structure and/or function of peptides but with modified backbone or side chains to enhance stability, bioavailability, or target specificity. They include peptoids, β-peptides, and other non-natural analogs.

Classification Based on Function:

Hormonal Peptides:

• Hormonal peptides are signaling molecules produced by endocrine glands or tissues that regulate various physiological processes. Examples include insulin (regulates glucose metabolism), oxytocin (regulates social bonding and childbirth), and growth hormone (regulates growth and metabolism).

Neuropeptides:

- Neuropeptides are peptides involved in signaling within the nervous system. They act as neurotransmitters, neuromodulators, or neurohormones, influencing behavior, pain perception, mood, and other neurological functions. Examples include endorphins, substance P, and neuropeptide Y.

Antimicrobial Peptides (AMPs):

- AMPs are peptides that have antimicrobial activity against bacteria, fungi, viruses, and parasites. They are part of the innate immune system and play a crucial role in defense against pathogens. Examples include defensins and cathelicidins.

Enzymatic Peptides:

- Enzymatic peptides act as catalysts in biochemical reactions, facilitating the breakdown of proteins (proteases), synthesis of peptides (peptidases), and other metabolic processes. Examples include trypsin, chymotrypsin, and pepsin.

Structural Peptides:

• Structural peptides contribute to the structural integrity of cells, tissues, and extracellular matrices. They include collagen (providing strength to connective tissues), elastin (providing elasticity), and keratin (providing strength to skin, hair, and nails).

Peptide Receptor Agonists/Antagonists:

• Peptides that bind to specific receptors on cell surfaces can act as agonists (activating receptors) or antagonists (blocking receptors), thereby regulating cellular signaling pathways. Examples include peptide hormone agonists (e.g., GLP-1 receptor agonists for diabetes treatment) and peptide antagonists (e.g., somatostatin analogs).

Combined Classification:

- Many peptides exhibit characteristics that can fit into multiple categories based on structure and function. For instance, insulin is both a hormonal peptide and a disulfide-bridged peptide. Understanding these classifications helps in studying their biological roles, designing therapeutic peptides, and exploring their potential applications in medicine and biotechnology.

CHAPTER TWO
Examples Of Therapeutic Peptide Families

Therapeutic peptides encompass a diverse range of families that have been developed for various medical applications. Here are some notable families of therapeutic peptides along with examples of their clinical uses:

Insulin and Analogues:

- **Insulin:** Used for the treatment of diabetes mellitus to regulate blood glucose levels.

- **Insulin Analogues (e.g., Lispro, Aspart, Glargine):** Modified forms of insulin with altered pharmacokinetic profiles to better mimic physiological insulin secretion.

Growth Hormone and Growth Hormone Releasing Peptides:

- **Growth Hormone (Somatropin):** Used to treat growth hormone deficiency in children and adults.

- **Growth Hormone Releasing Peptides (e.g., GHRP-2, GHRP-6):** Stimulate the release of growth hormone and are investigated for conditions like growth disorders and muscle wasting.

Glucagon-Like Peptide-1 (GLP-1) Agonists:

- **Exenatide, Liraglutide, Dulaglutide:** Used in the treatment of type 2 diabetes to improve glycemic control by stimulating insulin secretion and suppressing glucagon release.

Vasopressin and Analogs:

- **Desmopressin:** Used to treat diabetes insipidus and nocturnal enuresis.

- **Terlipressin:** Used for the treatment of hepatorenal syndrome and variceal bleeding.

Opioid Peptides and Analogs:

- **Morphine, Fentanyl, Buprenorphine:** Used for pain management due to their agonist activity on opioid receptors.

- **Endorphins:** Natural peptides with pain-relieving effects, studied for potential therapeutic applications.

Antimicrobial Peptides (AMPs):

- **Defensins (e.g., LL-37):** Natural peptides with broad-spectrum antimicrobial activity, investigated for treatment of infections.

- **Polymyxins (e.g., Colistin):** Peptide antibiotics used as a last resort for multidrug-resistant bacterial infections.

Somatostatin Analogs:

- **Octreotide, Lanreotide:** Used in the treatment of acromegaly, carcinoid syndrome, and certain types of tumors (e.g., neuroendocrine tumors) due to their ability to inhibit hormone secretion.

Enzyme Replacement Therapy (ERT) Peptides:

- **Laronidase, Imiglucerase:** Used to treat lysosomal storage disorders (e.g., Hurler syndrome, Gaucher disease) by replacing deficient enzymes.

Peptide Vaccines:

- **Synthetic Peptide Vaccines (e.g., HPV Peptide Vaccine):** Designed to induce immune responses against specific pathogens or tumor antigens, used in preventive and therapeutic vaccines.

Peptide Hormone Antagonists:

- **GnRH Antagonists (e.g., Degarelix):** Used in the treatment of prostate cancer by blocking gonadotropin-releasing hormone receptors, reducing testosterone levels.

These families of therapeutic peptides highlight their versatility in treating a wide range of medical conditions, from metabolic disorders and hormonal deficiencies to infectious diseases and cancer. Ongoing research continues to explore novel peptide-based therapies and improve existing treatments for better patient outcomes.

How Peptides Interact With Biological Targets

Peptides interact with biological targets through a variety of mechanisms, which depend on their structure, sequence, and the specific receptors or molecules they bind to. Understanding these interactions is crucial for developing peptide-based therapeutics and understanding their biological effects. Here are some key ways peptides interact with biological targets:

Receptor Binding:

• Many peptides exert their effects by binding to specific receptors on cell surfaces or within cells. These receptors are often proteins that recognize and bind to the peptide, triggering intracellular signaling pathways. Examples include peptide hormones like insulin binding to insulin receptors or neuropeptides binding to G-protein coupled receptors (GPCRs).

Enzyme Inhibition:

- Peptides can act as enzyme inhibitors by binding to and blocking the active sites of enzymes. This inhibition can disrupt biochemical pathways or regulatory processes. Examples include protease inhibitors, which block proteases involved in viral replication or protein degradation.

Ion Channel Modulation:

- Some peptides interact with ion channels, membrane proteins that regulate the flow of ions across cell membranes. By binding to ion channels, peptides can modulate their activity, affecting cellular excitability and neurotransmission. Examples include toxins from venomous animals that block or activate specific ion channels.

Transport Across Membranes:

- Certain peptides have the ability to cross cell membranes, either through passive diffusion or active transport mechanisms. Cell-penetrating peptides (CPPs) are examples of peptides that facilitate the delivery of cargo molecules (e.g., drugs, proteins) into cells, enhancing their therapeutic potential.

Protein-Protein Interactions:

• Peptides can interact with other proteins through specific binding interfaces, influencing protein-protein interactions critical for cellular signaling and regulation. Peptide inhibitors or mimetics can disrupt these interactions, potentially interfering with disease processes or regulatory pathways.

Structural Stability and Support:

• Structural peptides, such as collagen and elastin, provide structural stability and support to tissues. These peptides interact with other molecules (e.g., glycosaminoglycans) to form extracellular matrices that maintain tissue integrity and function.

Modulation of Gene Expression:

• Some peptides can regulate gene expression by interacting with transcription factors or other regulatory proteins. These interactions can influence cellular differentiation, proliferation, and responses to stimuli.

Immunological Interactions:

- Peptides play roles in immune responses by acting as antigens that elicit immune recognition and responses, or as antimicrobial peptides that directly kill pathogens. Peptide vaccines utilize this interaction to induce specific immune responses against pathogens or cancer cells.

These interactions highlight the diverse ways in which peptides contribute to biological functions and therapeutic effects. Understanding the mechanisms of peptide-target interactions is crucial for designing effective peptide-based drugs and therapies tailored to specific diseases and conditions.

CHAPTER THREE
Signaling Pathways And Cellular Responses

Peptides interact with biological systems through signaling pathways that orchestrate cellular responses. These pathways involve a series of molecular events triggered by peptide binding to receptors or other targets, leading to specific cellular responses. Here's an overview of how peptides participate in signaling pathways and induce cellular responses:

1. *Receptor-Mediated Signaling:*

• **Peptide Hormones:** Peptide hormones, such as insulin and glucagon, bind to specific receptors on cell surfaces. These receptors are often coupled to intracellular signaling pathways, such as the PI3K-Akt pathway or the MAPK pathway, which regulate processes like glucose uptake, metabolism, and gene expression.

- **Neuropeptides:** Neuropeptides interact with G-protein coupled receptors (GPCRs) in the nervous system. Activation of these receptors can modulate neurotransmitter release, neuronal excitability, and synaptic plasticity, influencing behaviors, mood, and pain perception.

2. Intracellular Signaling Pathways:

- **Second Messenger Systems:** Peptides can activate second messenger systems within cells. For example, cyclic AMP (cAMP) and calcium ions (Ca^{2+}) are common second messengers that relay signals from peptide receptors to downstream effectors, such as protein kinases and phosphatases.

- **Regulation of Gene Expression:** Certain peptides, like growth factors (e.g., EGF, TGF-β), can activate intracellular signaling pathways that regulate gene transcription. These pathways often involve the activation of transcription factors, which modulate the expression of genes involved in cell proliferation, differentiation, and survival.

3. Cellular Responses:

- **Metabolic Responses:** Peptides like insulin and glucagon regulate metabolic processes such as glucose uptake, glycogen synthesis, and lipid metabolism in response to changes in nutrient levels or physiological states.

- **Proliferation and Differentiation:** Growth factors and cytokines (e.g., EGF, PDGF) stimulate cell proliferation and differentiation by activating signaling pathways that promote cell cycle progression or induce changes in cellular morphology and function.

- **Apoptosis and Survival:** Peptides can influence cellular survival or programmed cell death (apoptosis). For instance, survival factors like Bcl-2 family proteins regulate apoptotic pathways, while cytokines such as TNF-α can trigger apoptosis under certain conditions.

- **Immune Responses:** Peptides participate in immune responses by regulating cytokine production, antigen presentation, and immune cell activation. They can act as chemotactic factors (e.g., chemokines) to recruit immune cells to sites of infection or inflammation.

4. Modulation of Cellular Function:

- **Neuronal Function:** Neuropeptides regulate neuronal excitability, synaptic transmission, and plasticity, influencing behaviors, learning, and memory.

- **Extracellular Matrix Dynamics:** Peptides like collagen and elastin peptides participate in maintaining the structural integrity of tissues and organs by influencing extracellular matrix remodeling and cell-matrix interactions.

5. Disease and Therapeutic Applications:

- Dysregulation of peptide signaling pathways is implicated in various diseases, including metabolic disorders (e.g., diabetes), cancer, neurodegenerative diseases, and autoimmune disorders.

- Peptide-based therapies target specific signaling pathways to modulate cellular responses, offering potential treatments for diseases characterized by aberrant peptide signaling or receptor function.

Peptides play crucial roles in cellular signaling pathways by binding to receptors, activating intracellular cascades, and orchestrating diverse cellular responses essential for physiological functions and disease processes. Understanding these pathways is fundamental for developing peptide-based drugs and therapies aimed at modulating cellular behavior and treating various medical conditions.

Methods For Designing Therapeutic Peptides

Designing therapeutic peptides involves several methods and approaches aimed at optimizing their stability, specificity, efficacy, and safety for clinical applications. Here are some key methods and strategies used in the design of therapeutic peptides:

1. Sequence Optimization:

- **Rational Design:** Involves designing peptides based on known receptor binding motifs or structural elements. This method uses computational tools to predict peptide-receptor interactions and optimize sequences for enhanced binding affinity and specificity.

- **Structure-Activity Relationship (SAR) Studies:** Experimentally assesses the impact of amino acid substitutions or modifications on peptide function. SAR studies help identify key residues critical for biological activity and improve peptide properties.

2. Modification and Cyclization:

- **Stabilization via Cyclization:** Cyclizing peptides by connecting the N- and C-termini or introducing disulfide bonds can enhance stability against proteolytic degradation and improve bioavailability.

- **Post-Translational Modifications (PTMs):** Incorporating PTMs like phosphorylation, glycosylation, or lipidation can modify peptide properties such as solubility, stability, or receptor affinity.

3. Peptide Mimetics:

- **Mimicking Peptide Structures:** Designing non-peptidic structures that mimic the biological activity of peptides while improving stability or pharmacokinetic properties. Examples include β-peptides or peptidomimetics with modified backbone structures.

4. Computational Modeling and Prediction:

- **Molecular Docking:** Using computational methods to predict peptide-receptor interactions and optimize binding affinity.

- **Quantitative Structure-Activity Relationship (QSAR):** Predicting peptide activity based on molecular descriptors and experimental data.

5. Bioconjugation and Delivery Systems:

- **Conjugation to Carriers:** Attaching peptides to carrier molecules (e.g., nanoparticles, liposomes) to improve stability, target specificity, and cellular uptake.

- **Cell-Penetrating Peptides (CPPs):** Incorporating CPPs to facilitate intracellular delivery of cargo molecules such as drugs or therapeutic proteins.

6. High-Throughput Screening:

- **Phage Display:** Screening peptide libraries displayed on bacteriophages to identify peptides that bind to specific targets or receptors.

- **Combinatorial Chemistry:** Synthesizing large libraries of peptides with diverse sequences to identify lead candidates with desired biological activities.

7. Targeted Therapeutic Applications:

- **Peptide Vaccines:** Designing peptides that mimic antigenic epitopes to induce specific immune responses against pathogens or cancer cells.

- **Peptide Inhibitors:** Developing peptides that antagonize receptor-ligand interactions or disrupt protein-protein interactions involved in disease pathways (e.g., enzyme inhibitors, receptor antagonists).

8. Validation and Optimization:

- **In vitro and in vivo Testing:** Evaluating the biological activity, stability, and toxicity of designed peptides using cell-based assays, animal models, and clinical trials.

- **Structure-Based Design:** Utilizing structural biology techniques such as X-ray crystallography or NMR spectroscopy to elucidate peptide-receptor interactions and guide rational design.

9. Safety and Pharmacokinetics:

- **Toxicity Assessment:** Evaluating potential cytotoxicity, immunogenicity, and off-target effects of therapeutic peptides.

- **Pharmacokinetic Optimization:** Modifying peptide properties (e.g., size, charge, hydrophobicity) to improve absorption, distribution, metabolism, and excretion (ADME) profiles.

10. Regulatory Considerations:

• **FDA Approval:** Ensuring compliance with regulatory guidelines for peptide-based therapeutics, including safety, efficacy, and manufacturing standards.

Designing therapeutic peptides involves an interdisciplinary approach combining molecular biology, chemistry, computational modeling, and pharmacology to create molecules with optimized therapeutic potential for treating various diseases and conditions.

CHAPTER FOUR
Techniques In Peptide Synthesis

Peptide synthesis refers to the process of creating peptides in the laboratory, either through solid-phase synthesis (SPPS) or liquid-phase synthesis. These techniques enable the production of peptides with precise sequences and functionalities, essential for both research and therapeutic applications. Here are the main techniques in peptide synthesis:

1. *Solid-Phase Peptide Synthesis (SPPS):*

• **Methodology:** SPPS is the most widely used method for peptide synthesis due to its efficiency and versatility. It involves building the peptide chain on a solid support (resin), typically with a derivatized polystyrene resin.

Process:

- **Activation:** The first amino acid is coupled to the resin via a linker. The amino acid is activated with a protecting group that reacts with the resin-bound linker.

- **Coupling:** Each subsequent amino acid is added sequentially, following activation with coupling reagents (e.g., DIC/HOBt or HBTU), forming peptide bonds between amino acids.

- **Deprotection:** After each coupling step, protecting groups are removed from the newly added amino acid to expose its reactive site for the next coupling.

- **Cleavage:** Upon completion of the peptide chain assembly, the peptide is cleaved from the resin and side chain protecting groups are removed.

- **Advantages:** Allows for stepwise synthesis of peptides with high purity and controlled sequence. Suitable for automated synthesis and synthesis of peptides with complex sequences.

- **Applications:** Used in pharmaceutical research, drug development, and biochemical studies to produce peptides ranging from small peptide hormones to larger proteins.

2. Liquid-Phase Peptide Synthesis:

- **Methodology:** Involves the direct chemical synthesis of peptides in solution phase, without the use of a solid support. It is typically used for shorter peptides or when solid-phase synthesis is not feasible.

- **Process:** Amino acids are sequentially coupled in solution using coupling reagents (e.g., carbodiimides), followed by deprotection steps to remove protecting groups.

- **Advantages:** Useful for synthesizing short peptides or peptides with challenging sequences. Allows for flexibility in peptide modification and optimization.

- **Applications:** Commonly used in peptide library synthesis, structure-activity relationship studies, and synthesis of peptide fragments for protein characterization.

3. Native Chemical Ligation (NCL):

- **Methodology:** NCL is a powerful method for synthesizing longer peptides and proteins by joining two unprotected peptide fragments under mild conditions.

- **Process:** Involves the reaction between a peptide fragment with a C-terminal thioester and another peptide fragment with an N-terminal cysteine or cysteine derivative. The reaction proceeds through a thioester exchange reaction followed by an S-N acyl shift to form a native peptide bond.

- **Advantages:** Enables synthesis of peptides and proteins with unnatural amino acids or modifications. Useful for synthesizing large and complex peptides that are challenging to produce by traditional methods.

- **Applications:** Used in chemical biology, protein engineering, and synthesis of therapeutic proteins or peptide-based drugs.

4. Hybrid Approaches and Modern Techniques:

- **Chemical Ligation Strategies:** Beyond NCL, other chemical ligation methods such as oxime ligation, hydrazone ligation, and Staudinger ligation are used for specific applications, including peptide-protein conjugation and modification.

- **Peptide Assembly:** Advances in peptide synthesis include combinatorial chemistry techniques, microwave-assisted synthesis, and automated synthesis platforms that improve efficiency, yield, and scalability of peptide production.

5. Post-Synthetic Modifications (PSMs):

- **Methodology:** After peptide synthesis, modifications such as conjugation with fluorophores, biotin, or other functional groups can be performed to enhance peptide properties or enable specific applications (e.g., peptide labeling for imaging studies).

- **Process:** Involves coupling of modified groups to peptide side chains or termini using coupling chemistries compatible with peptide stability and function.

- **Applications:** Widely used in biochemical and pharmaceutical research, as well as diagnostic and therapeutic applications requiring tailored peptide functionalities.

Each of these techniques in peptide synthesis offers unique advantages and applications, catering to the diverse needs of peptide-based research, drug development, and biotechnology. Advances in peptide synthesis continue to expand the capabilities and potential applications of peptides in biomedical sciences.

Challenges And Innovations In Peptide Delivery

Peptide delivery poses several challenges due to their inherent physicochemical properties, including poor stability, rapid degradation by proteases, and limited permeability across biological barriers.

Overcoming these challenges is crucial for enhancing the efficacy and therapeutic potential of peptide-based drugs. Here are some of the key challenges in peptide delivery and recent innovations aimed at addressing them:

Challenges in Peptide Delivery:

Proteolytic Degradation:

- Peptides are susceptible to degradation by proteases present in various tissues and bodily fluids, leading to reduced bioavailability and efficacy.

Poor Membrane Permeability:

- Peptides generally have low permeability across biological membranes, including the blood-brain barrier (BBB) and gastrointestinal (GI) tract, limiting their oral bioavailability and tissue penetration.

Short Half-Life:

- Rapid clearance from circulation due to enzymatic degradation and renal filtration results in short plasma half-lives for many peptides, necessitating frequent dosing or sustained-release formulations.

Immunogenicity and Toxicity:

- Some peptides may induce immune responses or exhibit cytotoxic effects, limiting their therapeutic application and safety profiles.

Specific Targeting:

• Achieving selective delivery to target tissues or cells while minimizing off-target effects remains a challenge, particularly for systemic administration.

Innovations in Peptide Delivery:

Modification and Conjugation Strategies:

- **PEGylation:** Conjugation of peptides with polyethylene glycol (PEG) can improve stability, prolong circulation half-life, and reduce immunogenicity by masking epitopes recognized by the immune system.

- **Lipidation:** Attachment of lipid moieties to peptides can enhance membrane permeability and cellular uptake, facilitating delivery across biological barriers.

- **Glycosylation:** Introducing glycosyl groups to peptides can improve stability and modify pharmacokinetic properties, reducing enzymatic degradation.

Nanoformulations:

- **Nanoparticles:** Encapsulation of peptides within nanoparticles (e.g., liposomes, polymeric nanoparticles) protects against enzymatic degradation, facilitates controlled release, and enhances targeting to specific tissues.

- **Micelles and Vesicles:** Self-assembling peptide-based structures like micelles and vesicles can encapsulate peptides and improve stability and bioavailability.

Cell-Penetrating Peptides (CPPs):

• CPPs are short peptides that facilitate cellular uptake of cargo molecules, including therapeutic peptides, through mechanisms such as direct translocation across membranes or endocytosis. CPPs can enhance delivery to intracellular targets.

Peptide-Protein Conjugates:

• Conjugation of peptides with proteins or antibodies can improve specificity and targeting to cell surface receptors or disease biomarkers, enhancing therapeutic efficacy while minimizing systemic exposure.

Sustained-Release Formulations:

• **Depot Injections:** Formulations designed for slow release of peptides from depot sites (e.g., subcutaneous or intramuscular injections) can extend dosing intervals and improve patient compliance.

• **Hydrogels and Implants:** Peptide-loaded hydrogels or implantable devices provide sustained release directly at the site of action, minimizing systemic exposure and enhancing therapeutic outcomes.

Innovative Administration Routes:

• **Inhalation and Intranasal Delivery:** Direct delivery of peptides to the lungs or nasal mucosa can bypass gastrointestinal degradation and achieve rapid absorption into systemic circulation or local tissues.

• **Topical and Transdermal Delivery:** Peptides formulated in creams, gels, or patches can penetrate through the skin barrier for localized treatment of skin disorders or systemic delivery.

Bioresponsive Delivery Systems:

- Smart delivery systems responsive to environmental cues (e.g., pH, enzymes) can release peptides selectively at disease sites or intracellular compartments, enhancing therapeutic efficacy and minimizing off-target effects.

Computational Design and Screening:

• Advances in computational modeling and high-throughput screening allow for the design and optimization of peptide sequences and delivery systems with improved stability, specificity, and pharmacokinetic profiles.

Ongoing innovations in peptide delivery aim to overcome the challenges associated with their physicochemical properties, enhancing their therapeutic potential across a wide range of diseases and conditions. Integration of these approaches continues to advance the field of peptide-based therapeutics, promising more effective and targeted treatments in the future.

CHAPTER FIVE
Routes Of Administration And Formulation Strategies

Peptides can be administered via various routes, each with specific formulation strategies tailored to optimize their delivery, bioavailability, and therapeutic efficacy. Here are the main routes of administration for peptides and corresponding formulation strategies:

Routes of Administration:

Parenteral Administration:

- **Subcutaneous Injection:** Peptides are injected into the layer of tissue just beneath the skin. This route allows for sustained release and is commonly used for peptides requiring gradual absorption into systemic circulation (e.g., insulin analogues for diabetes).

- **Formulation Strategies:** Formulate peptides as solutions or suspensions suitable for injection. Incorporate excipients to stabilize peptides, adjust pH, and enhance solubility.

- **Intramuscular Injection:** Peptides are injected directly into muscle tissue. This route allows for rapid absorption and is suitable for peptides with larger molecular sizes or when rapid onset of action is required.

- **Formulation Strategies:** Develop formulations that facilitate peptide dispersion and absorption in muscle tissue. Consider depot formulations for sustained release.

- **Intravenous Injection:** Peptides are administered directly into the bloodstream. This route provides immediate bioavailability and precise control over dosage.

- **Formulation Strategies:** Prepare peptides in sterile solutions compatible with intravenous administration. Ensure formulations are stable and free of particulates to prevent adverse reactions.

Oral Administration:

- **Oral Tablets/Capsules:** Peptides formulated as tablets or capsules for ingestion. This route offers convenience and patient compliance but faces challenges such as enzymatic degradation in the gastrointestinal (GI) tract and poor oral bioavailability due to low membrane permeability.

- **Formulation Strategies:** Enhance stability against GI enzymes using enteric coatings or enzyme inhibitors. Utilize absorption enhancers or prodrug approaches to improve membrane permeability and absorption.

- **Oral Dispersible Formulations:** Peptides formulated as powders or lyophilized formulations that dissolve or disperse quickly in saliva for absorption through the oral mucosa.

- **Formulation Strategies:** Incorporate mucoadhesive polymers or permeation enhancers to facilitate absorption through the buccal or sublingual mucosa. Ensure stability and rapid dissolution characteristics.

Pulmonary Administration:

- **Inhalation:** Peptides delivered via inhalation as aerosols or dry powder formulations. This route targets the respiratory tract for local or systemic effects, bypassing GI degradation and achieving rapid absorption.

- **Formulation Strategies:** Develop inhalable formulations with appropriate particle size for deposition in the lungs. Stabilize peptides against aerosolization stresses and ensure compatibility with inhalation devices.

Transdermal Administration:

• **Topical Applications:** Peptides formulated in creams, gels, or patches for application to the skin. This route enables localized treatment of dermatological conditions or systemic delivery.

• **Formulation Strategies:** Optimize formulations for skin permeability and absorption. Use penetration enhancers or nanocarriers to facilitate peptide transport across the skin barrier.

Nasal Administration:

• **Intranasal Spray:** Peptides administered via nasal sprays or drops. This route allows for rapid absorption into systemic circulation through nasal mucosa, bypassing first-pass metabolism.

• **Formulation Strategies:** Develop formulations with appropriate pH and osmolarity for nasal tolerance. Enhance peptide stability and absorption using mucoadhesive agents or permeation enhancers.

Formulation Strategies:

- **Stabilization:** Protect peptides from enzymatic degradation using enzyme inhibitors or modifying peptide sequences for stability.

- **Solubility Enhancement:** Use solubilizers, co-solvents, or pH adjustments to improve peptide solubility and formulation compatibility.

- **Targeting and Release:** Incorporate targeting ligands or stimuli-responsive materials to achieve site-specific delivery or controlled release of peptides.

- **Encapsulation:** Use nanocarriers (e.g., liposomes, nanoparticles) to encapsulate peptides, protecting them from degradation and facilitating controlled release.

- **Sustained Release:** Develop sustained-release formulations (e.g., depot injections, implants) to prolong peptide activity and reduce dosing frequency.

- **Safety and Biocompatibility:** Ensure formulations are biocompatible, sterile, and free from contaminants or allergens to minimize adverse effects.

- **Regulatory Considerations:** Comply with regulatory guidelines for pharmaceutical formulation, ensuring stability, efficacy, and safety of peptide-based products.

Each route of administration and corresponding formulation strategy presents unique opportunities and challenges for delivering peptides effectively in therapeutic applications. Advances in formulation technology continue to expand the possibilities for optimizing peptide delivery, enhancing their clinical utility in treating various diseases and conditions.

Applications Of Peptide Therapy For Alzheimer's, Parkinson's, Etc.

Peptide therapy holds promise in the treatment of neurodegenerative diseases like Alzheimer's disease (AD) and Parkinson's disease (PD) due to its potential to target specific pathological mechanisms and improve therapeutic outcomes. Here are some key applications and strategies for peptide therapy in these neurodegenerative conditions:

Alzheimer's Disease (AD):

Amyloid Beta (Aβ) Aggregation Inhibitors:

- **Target:** Aβ peptides play a central role in the formation of amyloid plaques, a hallmark of AD pathology.

- **Peptide Therapy:** Peptides designed to inhibit Aβ aggregation or promote its clearance have been investigated. For example, β-sheet breaker peptides can disrupt Aβ aggregation, potentially slowing disease progression.

Tau Protein Modulators:

- **Target:** Abnormal phosphorylation and aggregation of tau protein contribute to neurofibrillary tangle formation in AD.

- **Peptide Therapy:** Peptides targeting tau phosphorylation sites or stabilizing tau conformation may prevent or reduce tau aggregation. Tau-based immunotherapies using peptide epitopes are also being explored.

Neuroprotective Peptides:

- **Target:** Protecting neurons from oxidative stress, inflammation, and excitotoxicity, which contribute to neuronal damage in AD.

- **Peptide Therapy:** Peptides with antioxidant, anti-inflammatory, or neurotrophic properties aim to enhance neuronal survival and function. Examples include brain-derived neurotrophic factor (BDNF) mimetics or neurotrophic factor-derived peptides.

Blood-Brain Barrier (BBB) Penetration:

- **Challenge:** Peptides must cross the BBB to exert therapeutic effects in the brain.

- **Peptide Therapy:** Utilizing cell-penetrating peptides (CPPs) or peptide carriers that facilitate BBB penetration can enhance delivery of therapeutic peptides to the brain parenchyma.

Immunomodulatory Peptides:

- **Target:** Modulating immune responses implicated in AD pathogenesis, including neuroinflammation and microglial activation.

- **Peptide Therapy:** Peptides targeting immune receptors or inflammatory mediators may attenuate neuroinflammation and support neuronal function.

Parkinson's Disease (PD):

Alpha-Synuclein Aggregation Inhibitors:

- **Target:** Alpha-synuclein (α-syn) aggregation and accumulation in Lewy bodies are characteristic of PD.

- **Peptide Therapy:** Peptides designed to inhibit α-syn aggregation or promote its clearance are under investigation. These peptides may prevent neurotoxicity associated with α-syn aggregates.

Dopaminergic Neuron Protection:

- **Target:** Preservation of dopaminergic neurons in the substantia nigra, whose degeneration leads to motor symptoms in PD.

- **Peptide Therapy:** Peptides with neuroprotective properties, such as antioxidants or growth factors promoting dopaminergic neuron survival, are being explored.

Mitochondrial Function Modulators:

• **Target:** Enhancing mitochondrial function and reducing oxidative stress, which contribute to neuronal degeneration in PD.

• **Peptide Therapy:** Peptides targeting mitochondrial dysfunction or promoting mitochondrial biogenesis may mitigate neurodegeneration and improve cellular energy metabolism.

Neurotrophic Factor Delivery:

- **Target:** Supporting neuronal survival and function in PD-afflicted regions of the brain.

- **Peptide Therapy:** Peptides mimicking or delivering neurotrophic factors like glial cell-derived neurotrophic factor (GDNF) or brain-derived neurotrophic factor (BDNF) could promote neuroprotection and regeneration of dopaminergic neurons.

Gene Therapy Delivery Vectors:

- **Approach:** Peptide carriers or vectors for delivering gene therapy constructs (e.g., viral vectors, nucleic acids) aimed at modifying disease progression or promoting neuroprotective pathways in PD.

Clinical Challenges and Considerations:

- **BBB Permeability:** Developing strategies to enhance peptide delivery across the BBB is crucial for effective treatment of neurodegenerative diseases.

- **Safety and Immunogenicity:** Peptides must be designed to minimize immunogenicity and potential side effects, ensuring safety in chronic treatment regimens.

- **Target Specificity:** Achieving selective targeting of pathological proteins or cells while sparing healthy tissues is essential to maximize therapeutic efficacy.

- **Combination Therapies:** Investigating synergistic effects of peptide therapy with existing treatments (e.g., small molecule drugs, immunotherapy) to optimize therapeutic outcomes and disease management.

Peptide therapy offers diverse strategies for targeting underlying mechanisms of neurodegenerative diseases like Alzheimer's and Parkinson's, holding potential for disease-modifying treatments that improve patient outcomes and quality of life. Continued research and clinical trials are essential to validate these approaches and advance peptide-based therapies towards clinical application.

CHAPTER SIX
Neuroprotective Peptides And Their Mechanisms

Neuroprotective peptides are a class of molecules that demonstrate the ability to protect neurons from various forms of damage and degeneration, making them promising candidates for therapeutic applications in neurodegenerative diseases and neurological disorders.

These peptides exert their effects through several mechanisms, each contributing to neuronal survival, function, and resilience against pathological insults.

Here are some neuroprotective peptides and their mechanisms of action:

1. Brain-Derived Neurotrophic Factor (BDNF) and Derived Peptides:

- **Mechanism:** BDNF is a neurotrophin that promotes neuronal survival, differentiation, and synaptic plasticity. Peptides derived from BDNF or mimicking its active domains can mimic these neurotrophic effects.

Actions:

- **Neuroprotection:** Enhances survival of neurons under stress conditions.

- **Synaptic Plasticity:** Promotes formation and strengthening of synaptic connections.

- **Neurogenesis:** Stimulates generation of new neurons in the brain.

- **Clinical Relevance:** Implicated in conditions such as Alzheimer's disease, Parkinson's disease, and stroke, where BDNF deficiency or dysfunction contributes to neuronal degeneration.

2. Glial Cell-Derived Neurotrophic Factor (GDNF) and Mimetics:

- **Mechanism:** GDNF is another neurotrophic factor that supports the survival and function of dopaminergic neurons in the substantia nigra.

Actions:

- **Dopaminergic Neuron Protection:** Protects dopaminergic neurons from degeneration in Parkinson's disease.

- **Neuroregeneration:** Promotes axonal growth and neuronal repair.

- **Clinical Relevance:** Investigated for its potential in Parkinson's disease treatment to mitigate motor symptoms and slow disease progression.

3. Peptides Targeting Oxidative Stress and Mitochondrial Function:

- **Mechanism:** Many neurodegenerative diseases involve oxidative stress and mitochondrial dysfunction, leading to neuronal damage and death. Peptides targeting these pathways can provide neuroprotection.

Actions:

- **Antioxidant Activity:** Scavenge free radicals and reduce oxidative damage to neurons.

- **Mitochondrial Protection:** Maintain mitochondrial function and biogenesis.

- **Examples:** Peptides like SS-31 (Bendavia) that target mitochondrial membranes to preserve their integrity and function.

4. Anti-Inflammatory and Immunomodulatory Peptides:

- **Mechanism:** Chronic inflammation and immune activation contribute to neurodegeneration. Peptides modulating immune responses and inflammation can protect neurons from inflammatory damage.

Actions:

- **Anti-Inflammatory Effects:** Suppress cytokine production and microglial activation.

- **Immunomodulation:** Regulate immune responses to reduce neuroinflammation.

- **Examples:** Neuropeptides or synthetic peptides that inhibit inflammatory pathways or modulate immune cell function.

5. Peptides Modulating Apoptotic Pathways:

- **Mechanism:** Apoptosis (programmed cell death) pathways are dysregulated in neurodegenerative diseases. Peptides targeting apoptotic pathways can prevent neuronal cell death.

Actions:

- **Anti-Apoptotic Effects:** Inhibit caspase activation and promote cell survival signals.

- **Cell Survival Promotion:** Maintain cellular integrity and function under stress conditions.

- **Examples:** Peptides derived from endogenous anti-apoptotic proteins or designed to mimic their protective actions.

6. Neurotensin and Neurotensin Receptor Agonists:

- **Mechanism:** Neurotensin is a neuropeptide involved in modulating dopamine signaling and has neuroprotective properties.

Actions:

- **Neuroprotection:** Protects neurons from oxidative stress and excitotoxicity.

- **Neurotransmitter Regulation:** Modulates dopamine release and neurotransmitter balance.

- **Clinical Relevance:** Investigated for potential therapeutic applications in Parkinson's disease and other neurodegenerative disorders affecting dopamine pathways.

Clinical and Therapeutic Applications:

- **Stroke Recovery:** Peptides promoting neuronal survival and regeneration are explored for enhancing recovery post-stroke.

- **Neurodegenerative Diseases:** Peptide-based therapies are investigated for their potential to slow disease progression and improve symptoms in Alzheimer's, Parkinson's, and Huntington's diseases.

- **Traumatic Brain Injury:** Neuroprotective peptides are studied for their ability to mitigate secondary injury processes and promote neural repair after traumatic brain injury.

Neuroprotective peptides exert their effects through diverse mechanisms, including neurotrophic support, antioxidant properties, modulation of inflammatory responses, and regulation of apoptotic pathways. Continued research and clinical trials are essential to validate these peptides as safe and effective therapies for neurodegenerative diseases and other neurological conditions.

Peptide Hormones In Diabetes Management

Peptide hormones play crucial roles in diabetes management, influencing glucose metabolism, insulin secretion, and overall metabolic homeostasis. Here are some key peptide hormones involved in diabetes and their roles in management:

1. Insulin:

• **Role:** Insulin is a peptide hormone produced by pancreatic beta cells in response to elevated blood glucose levels.

• **Function:** It facilitates glucose uptake into cells, promotes glycogen synthesis in the liver and muscles, and inhibits gluconeogenesis, thereby lowering blood glucose levels.

- **Clinical Use:** Insulin therapy is essential for managing type 1 diabetes mellitus (T1DM) and may be required in advanced stages of type 2 diabetes mellitus (T2DM) when oral medications are insufficient.

2. Glucagon:

- **Role:** Glucagon is a peptide hormone produced by pancreatic alpha cells in response to low blood glucose levels.

- **Function:** It stimulates glycogen breakdown (glycogenolysis) and gluconeogenesis in the liver, leading to an increase in blood glucose levels.

- **Clinical Use:** Glucagon is used in emergency kits for severe hypoglycemia (low blood sugar) in patients with diabetes who are unable to consume glucose orally.

3. Glucagon-Like Peptide-1 (GLP-1):

• **Role:** GLP-1 is an incretin hormone released from intestinal L cells in response to food intake.

• **Function:** It enhances glucose-dependent insulin secretion, suppresses glucagon secretion, slows gastric emptying, and promotes satiety.

• **Clinical Use:** GLP-1 receptor agonists (e.g., exenatide, liraglutide) are used as injectable therapies for T2DM to improve glycemic control, reduce weight, and lower cardiovascular risk.

4. Glucose-Dependent Insulinotropic Peptide (GIP):

- **Role:** GIP is another incretin hormone released from intestinal K cells in response to nutrient ingestion.

- **Function:** It stimulates insulin secretion in a glucose-dependent manner, inhibits glucagon release, and promotes fat storage.

- **Clinical Use:** GIP receptor agonists are being investigated as potential therapies for T2DM, although none are currently approved for clinical use.

5. Amylin:

- **Role:** Amylin is a peptide co-secreted with insulin from pancreatic beta cells.

- **Function:** It regulates postprandial glucose levels by suppressing glucagon secretion, slowing gastric emptying, and promoting satiety.

- **Clinical Use:** Pramlintide, a synthetic analog of amylin, is used as an adjunct therapy in T1DM and T2DM to improve glycemic control, especially postprandial glucose levels.

6. Adiponectin:

- **Role:** Adiponectin is a peptide hormone produced by adipose tissue.

- **Function:** It enhances insulin sensitivity, promotes fatty acid oxidation, and reduces inflammation.

- **Clinical Relevance:** Low levels of adiponectin are associated with insulin resistance and T2DM. Strategies to increase adiponectin levels may have therapeutic potential in diabetes management.

Therapeutic Applications and Considerations:

- **Combination Therapies:** Peptide hormones are often used in combination with oral antidiabetic medications (e.g., metformin, sulfonylureas) or insulin therapy to achieve optimal glycemic control in diabetes patients.

- **Route of Administration:** While insulin is typically administered via subcutaneous injection, GLP-1 receptor agonists and amylin analogs are also available as injectable formulations. Efforts are ongoing to develop alternative delivery methods (e.g., oral formulations, inhalable peptides) to improve patient adherence and convenience.

- **Emerging Therapies:** Ongoing research focuses on developing novel peptide-based therapies targeting pathways such as GIP receptors, adiponectin modulation, and dual or triple agonists targeting multiple metabolic pathways.

Peptide hormones play critical roles in glucose metabolism and diabetes management, with therapeutic strategies evolving to enhance efficacy, safety, and patient compliance in treating both T1DM and T2DM.

CHAPTER SEVEN
Growth Hormone Therapies And Beyond

Growth hormone (GH) therapies have evolved significantly beyond their initial use in treating growth disorders to encompass a wide range of therapeutic applications in various medical conditions. Here's an overview of growth hormone therapies and their broader applications:

Growth Hormone Therapy

Treatment of Growth Disorders:

- **Role:** Growth hormone is essential for stimulating growth and development in children and adolescents.

- **Indications:** GH therapy is primarily used to treat growth hormone deficiency (GHD), Turner syndrome, chronic kidney disease (CKD) causing growth failure, and Prader-Willi syndrome.

- **Administration:** Typically administered via daily subcutaneous injections.

Adult Growth Hormone Deficiency:

- **Role:** GH deficiency in adults can lead to metabolic abnormalities, reduced bone density, and impaired quality of life.

- **Indications:** GH therapy in adults with GHD is used to improve body composition, muscle mass, bone density, and overall well-being.

Athletic Performance and Bodybuilding:

• **Role:** Despite controversial use, GH has been abused for its purported performance-enhancing effects in athletes and bodybuilders.

• **Concerns:** Misuse can lead to serious health risks, including cardiovascular complications, joint disorders, and metabolic disturbances.

Beyond Growth Hormone: Therapeutic Applications

Metabolic Disorders:

• **Role:** GH plays a crucial role in metabolism, influencing lipid metabolism, insulin sensitivity, and glucose homeostasis.

• **Indications:** GH therapy is explored in conditions such as lipodystrophy, where it can improve lipid profiles and metabolic parameters.

Osteoporosis and Bone Health:

- **Role:** GH contributes to bone metabolism and mineralization.

- **Indications:** GH therapy may benefit patients with osteoporosis or bone fractures by promoting bone formation and reducing fracture risk.

Anti-Aging and Longevity:

- **Role:** GH has been associated with anti-aging effects, including improved skin elasticity, muscle mass maintenance, and cognitive function.

- **Controversy:** Long-term safety and efficacy for anti-aging purposes are debated, and GH therapy for anti-aging is not approved by regulatory agencies.

Cachexia and Muscle Wasting Disorders:

- **Role:** GH promotes muscle protein synthesis and inhibits protein breakdown.

- **Indications:** GH therapy is investigated in conditions associated with muscle wasting, such as HIV/AIDS-related cachexia and chronic obstructive pulmonary disease (COPD).

Psychiatric Disorders:

- **Role:** GH and its receptors are present in the central nervous system, influencing mood, cognition, and neuroprotection.

- **Indications:** GH therapy is being explored in psychiatric disorders such as depression and cognitive decline associated with aging.

Innovations and Future Directions

Long-Acting GH Formulations:

- **Role:** Development of long-acting GH formulations aims to improve treatment adherence and reduce injection frequency.

- **Examples:** Pegylated GH formulations with extended half-lives are in clinical development.

GH Receptor Agonists and Antagonists:

- **Role:** Novel compounds targeting GH receptors are being developed to modulate GH signaling pathways with potential applications in metabolic disorders and aging-related conditions.

Combination Therapies:

- **Role:** Integration of GH therapy with other hormonal therapies or pharmacological agents to optimize therapeutic outcomes and address multiple facets of complex conditions.

Biomarkers and Personalized Medicine:

- **Role:** Advances in biomarker research may enable personalized GH therapy based on individual metabolic and genetic profiles, improving treatment efficacy and safety.

Considerations and Challenges:

- **Safety Concerns:** Long-term safety of GH therapy, particularly in non-GHD conditions, requires careful monitoring due to potential risks such as glucose intolerance, cardiovascular effects, and tumor growth.

- **Regulatory Approval:** GH therapies for non-traditional indications often face regulatory scrutiny and require robust clinical evidence of efficacy and safety.

- **Ethical and Legal Issues:** Off-label use and abuse of GH for performance enhancement raise ethical and legal concerns, emphasizing the need for responsible prescribing practices and regulatory oversight.

Growth hormone therapies have expanded beyond their traditional use in growth disorders to encompass diverse therapeutic applications in metabolic disorders, bone health, muscle wasting conditions, and potentially psychiatric disorders and anti-aging.

Ongoing research and technological advancements aim to optimize the efficacy, safety, and accessibility of GH therapies across various medical contexts.

Peptide Vaccines And Immune Modulation

Peptide vaccines represent a novel approach to vaccination that utilizes synthetic peptides derived from specific antigens to induce targeted immune responses against pathogens or cancer cells. These vaccines leverage peptide fragments that mimic the epitopes recognized by the immune system, aiming to elicit protective immunity or therapeutic responses. Here's how peptide vaccines work and their role in immune modulation:

Mechanism of Action

Antigen Presentation:

- Peptide vaccines consist of short peptide sequences that mimic antigenic epitopes derived from pathogens or tumor antigens.

- Antigen-presenting cells (APCs), such as dendritic cells, process and present these peptides via major histocompatibility complex (MHC) molecules to T cells.

T Cell Activation:

- Peptide-MHC complexes on APCs interact with T cell receptors (TCRs) on CD4+ T helper cells or CD8+ cytotoxic T cells.

- This interaction triggers T cell activation, leading to the proliferation and differentiation of antigen-specific T cells.

Immune Response Initiation:

- Activated CD4+ T cells help in B cell activation and antibody production (humoral immunity).

- Activated CD8+ T cells recognize and kill infected cells or tumor cells presenting the peptide antigens (cell-mediated immunity).

Memory Response:

- Successful vaccination with peptide antigens results in the generation of memory T cells that can rapidly respond to future encounters with the pathogen or tumor antigens.

Immune Modulation

Enhancing Immune Response:

• Peptide vaccines can be designed to enhance specific immune responses against pathogens or cancer cells by targeting unique epitopes.

• They can induce robust T cell responses, particularly cytotoxic T lymphocytes (CTLs), which are crucial for eliminating infected or malignant cells.

Reducing Autoimmunity:

• Peptide vaccines can also modulate immune responses to prevent or attenuate autoimmune diseases by inducing immune tolerance or regulatory T cell responses.

• They may target specific autoantigens involved in autoimmune processes to induce immune deviation or tolerance.

Precision Medicine Approach:

- Peptide vaccines allow for personalized medicine approaches, where vaccine antigens can be selected based on individual tumor or pathogen profiles.

- This precision targeting enhances vaccine efficacy and reduces off-target effects compared to traditional broad-spectrum vaccines.

Clinical Applications

Infectious Diseases:

Peptide vaccines are under investigation for preventing infections such as influenza, hepatitis B, human papillomavirus (HPV), and malaria.

- They offer potential advantages like enhanced safety profiles and the ability to incorporate multiple antigens for broader protection.

Cancer Immunotherapy:

- Peptide vaccines are being explored as cancer immunotherapies to target tumor-specific antigens.

- Examples include vaccines against melanoma-associated antigens (e.g., gp100, MART-1) or neoantigens derived from mutated proteins in individual tumors.

Autoimmune Diseases:

- Peptide vaccines hold promise for inducing antigen-specific tolerance in autoimmune diseases like multiple sclerosis, type 1 diabetes, and rheumatoid arthritis.

- They aim to suppress pathological immune responses while preserving protective immunity against infections.

Challenges and Future Directions

- **Antigen Selection:** Identifying optimal peptide antigens that induce strong and durable immune responses remains a challenge.

- **Delivery Systems:** Developing effective delivery systems to enhance peptide stability, immunogenicity, and uptake by APCs is crucial for vaccine efficacy.

- **Adjuvants:** Incorporating adjuvants or immune stimulants to enhance peptide vaccine potency and duration of immune responses.

- **Clinical Validation:** Conducting robust clinical trials to demonstrate safety, efficacy, and long-term benefits of peptide vaccines in diverse populations and disease contexts.

Peptide vaccines represent a promising approach for immune modulation against infectious diseases, cancer, and autoimmune disorders.

Advances in peptide design, delivery technologies, and immunological understanding are expected to drive further innovation and clinical application of peptide-based vaccination strategies.

CHAPTER EIGHT
Applications In Autoimmune Diseases

Peptide-based therapies show considerable promise in the treatment of autoimmune diseases, leveraging their ability to modulate immune responses towards self-antigens while preserving overall immune function. Here are some key applications and strategies of peptide-based therapies in autoimmune diseases:

Mechanisms of Action

Induction of Tolerance:

- **Role:** Peptide vaccines or therapies can induce antigen-specific tolerance, suppressing autoimmune responses against self-antigens.

- **Mechanism:** Administration of peptides derived from autoantigens can induce regulatory T cells (Tregs) or anergy in autoreactive T cells, leading to immune tolerance.

Modulation of Immune Response:

- **Role:** Peptides can modulate immune responses by targeting specific immune receptors or signaling pathways involved in autoimmune pathology.

- **Mechanism:** Peptides may act as agonists or antagonists to influence cytokine production, T cell activation, or B cell responses critical in autoimmune diseases.

Applications in Specific Autoimmune Diseases

Multiple Sclerosis (MS):

- **Target:** Myelin-derived peptides (e.g., myelin basic protein, myelin oligodendrocyte glycoprotein) implicated in MS pathogenesis.

- **Approach:** Peptide therapies aim to induce immune tolerance to myelin antigens, reducing autoimmune attack on the central nervous system.

Type 1 Diabetes (T1D):

- **Target:** Pancreatic islet antigens such as insulin or glutamic acid decarboxylase (GAD65).

- **Approach:** Peptide vaccines or therapies seek to suppress autoreactive T cells targeting insulin-producing beta cells, preserving insulin secretion.

Rheumatoid Arthritis (RA):

• **Target:** Peptides derived from joint-specific antigens like type II collagen or citrullinated peptides.

• **Approach:** Peptide-based therapies aim to induce tolerance to joint-specific antigens, reducing inflammation and joint damage.

Celiac Disease:

• **Target:** Gluten-derived peptides that trigger immune responses in individuals with celiac disease.

• **Approach:** Peptide therapies may induce immune tolerance to gluten peptides, preventing intestinal inflammation and damage.

Clinical Trials and Developments

Antigen-Specific Immunotherapy:

- **Approach:** Clinical trials are investigating peptide-based vaccines or oral formulations targeting specific autoantigens in autoimmune diseases.

- **Examples:** Trials for T1D focus on proinsulin or GAD65 peptides, while MS trials may target myelin peptides.

Immune Modulation Strategies:

- **Approach:** Combining peptides with adjuvants or immune modulators to enhance therapeutic efficacy and induce durable immune tolerance.

- **Examples:** Use of tolerogenic nanoparticles or cytokine modulators alongside peptide therapies in autoimmune diseases.

Challenges and Considerations

- **Antigen Selection:** Identifying the most relevant and immunogenic peptide antigens for each autoimmune disease presents a challenge.

- **Safety and Tolerability:** Ensuring peptide therapies induce antigen-specific tolerance without compromising overall immune function or increasing infection risks.

- **Individualized Treatment:** Developing personalized peptide therapies based on patient-specific immune profiles and disease heterogeneity.

- **Regulatory Approval:** Establishing robust clinical evidence to support regulatory approval and widespread adoption of peptide-based therapies in autoimmune diseases.

In summary, peptide-based therapies hold significant potential for inducing immune tolerance and modulating autoimmune responses in diseases like MS, T1D, RA, and others. Ongoing research aims to refine peptide design, delivery methods, and combination therapies to optimize efficacy and safety in treating autoimmune disorders.

Peptides In Targeted Cancer Therapies

Peptides are increasingly being explored as targeted therapies for cancer due to their specificity, potency, and potential for minimal off-target effects compared to traditional chemotherapy. Here's an overview of how peptides are utilized in targeted cancer therapies:

Mechanisms of Action

Targeting Cancer Cell Surface Receptors:

- **Role:** Peptides can be designed to specifically target receptors overexpressed on cancer cell surfaces.

- **Mechanism:** Upon binding to these receptors, peptide conjugates or peptides themselves can induce cytotoxicity or inhibit signaling pathways crucial for cancer cell survival and proliferation.

Inhibition of Protein-Protein Interactions:

- **Role:** Peptides can disrupt critical protein-protein interactions (PPIs) involved in cancer progression.

- **Mechanism:** Peptides mimic binding motifs of interacting proteins, thereby preventing formation of complexes essential for cancer cell survival or metastasis.

Induction of Apoptosis:

- **Role:** Some peptides are designed to penetrate cancer cells and induce programmed cell death (apoptosis).

- **Mechanism:** These peptides may target mitochondrial membranes, activate caspases, or interfere with survival pathways, leading to cancer cell death.

Drug Delivery Vehicles:

- **Role:** Peptides can serve as carriers for delivering cytotoxic drugs, radionuclides, or imaging agents directly to cancer cells.

- **Mechanism:** Peptide-drug conjugates or nanoparticles conjugated with targeting peptides enhance specificity and reduce systemic toxicity.

Types of Peptides in Targeted Cancer Therapies

Antibody-Derived Peptides:

- **Role:** Peptides derived from monoclonal antibodies (mAbs) targeting cancer-specific antigens.

- **Mechanism:** These peptides retain specificity for cancer cells while potentially improving tissue penetration and reducing immunogenicity compared to full-length antibodies.

Cell-Penetrating Peptides (CPPs):

- **Role:** Short peptides capable of crossing cell membranes.

- **Mechanism:** CPPs deliver cytotoxic drugs or therapeutic cargoes directly into cancer cells, enhancing drug efficacy and reducing systemic side effects.

Peptide Hormones and Receptors:

- **Role:** Peptide hormones or receptor-targeting peptides implicated in cancer growth regulation.

- **Mechanism:** Targeting receptors such as growth hormone receptors or peptide hormone receptors on cancer cells can disrupt signaling pathways or deliver therapeutic payloads.

Peptide Vaccines and Immunotherapy:

- **Role:** Peptides derived from tumor-associated antigens (TAAs) or neoantigens.

- **Mechanism:** Peptide vaccines stimulate the immune system to recognize and attack cancer cells presenting specific antigens, promoting immune-mediated tumor regression.

Clinical Applications and Developments

Targeted Therapy Approvals:

- **Examples:** FDA-approved peptide-based therapies include somatostatin analogs (e.g., octreotide) for neuroendocrine tumors and peptide receptor radionuclide therapy (PRRT) for neuroendocrine cancers and certain types of metastatic tumors.

Emerging Peptide Targets:

- **Examples:** Peptides targeting integrins, growth factor receptors (EGFR, HER2), and vascular endothelial growth factor (VEGF) receptors are under investigation in clinical trials for various cancers.

Combination Therapies:

- **Approach:** Integrating peptide-based therapies with traditional chemotherapy, radiotherapy, or immunotherapy to enhance treatment outcomes and overcome resistance mechanisms in cancer.

Challenges and Future Directions

- **Peptide Stability:** Enhancing peptide stability against enzymatic degradation and optimizing pharmacokinetics for improved efficacy.

- **Tumor Penetration:** Overcoming barriers to efficient peptide delivery and penetration into solid tumors to reach cancer cells effectively.

- **Resistance Mechanisms:** Understanding and addressing mechanisms of resistance to peptide therapies, such as downregulation of target receptors or acquired mutations.

- **Personalized Medicine:** Developing personalized peptide therapies based on tumor-specific biomarkers or genetic profiles to maximize therapeutic response.

Peptides hold significant promise in targeted cancer therapies by leveraging their specificity and diverse mechanisms of action. Ongoing research and clinical trials are expected to advance peptide-based treatments, potentially transforming cancer treatment paradigms with enhanced efficacy and reduced toxicity.

CHAPTER NINE
Tumor Targeting And Anti-Angiogenic Peptides

Tumor targeting and anti-angiogenic peptides represent innovative strategies in cancer therapy, aiming to selectively target cancer cells or disrupt the formation of new blood vessels crucial for tumor growth and metastasis. Here's an overview of these approaches:

Tumor Targeting Peptides

Tumor targeting peptides are designed to specifically recognize and bind to molecules or receptors overexpressed on the surface of cancer cells. This targeted approach enhances the specificity of therapy, potentially minimizing damage to healthy tissues.

Here are key aspects of tumor targeting peptides:

Peptide Selection Criteria:

• Peptides are selected based on their ability to bind selectively to tumor-specific antigens or receptors.

• Common targets include receptors overexpressed on cancer cells, such as integrins (e.g., $\alpha v\beta 3$, $\alpha v\beta 5$), growth factor receptors (e.g., EGFR, HER2), or tumor-specific antigens.

Mechanisms of Action:

• **Direct Cytotoxicity:** Some peptides are designed to induce apoptosis or disrupt signaling pathways specific to cancer cells upon binding.

• **Drug Delivery:** Peptides can serve as carriers for delivering cytotoxic drugs, radionuclides, or imaging agents directly to tumors, enhancing therapeutic efficacy and reducing systemic toxicity.

- **Immunotherapy:** Peptide vaccines targeting tumor-associated antigens (TAAs) can stimulate immune responses against cancer cells, promoting tumor regression through immune-mediated mechanisms.

Examples of Targeted Peptides:

- **RGD Peptides:** Recognize integrins overexpressed on tumor vasculature and cancer cells, facilitating tumor homing and delivery of therapeutic payloads.

- **Somatostatin Analogues:** Target receptors overexpressed in neuroendocrine tumors, used in peptide receptor radionuclide therapy (PRRT) for targeted treatment.

- **Epidermal Growth Factor (EGF) Peptides:** Bind to EGFR overexpressed in various cancers, facilitating targeted drug delivery or immunotherapy.

Anti-Angiogenic Peptides

- Anti-angiogenic peptides inhibit the process of angiogenesis, which is crucial for tumor growth and metastasis by promoting the formation of new blood vessels from existing vasculature. Here's how anti-angiogenic peptides function:

Mechanisms of Anti-Angiogenic Action:

- **Inhibition of Growth Factors:** Peptides can block vascular endothelial growth factor (VEGF) receptors or other angiogenic growth factor receptors, inhibiting endothelial cell proliferation and angiogenesis.

- **Disruption of Vessel Formation:** Peptides may interfere with endothelial cell migration, tube formation, or vessel stabilization critical for tumor vascularization.

Applications in Cancer Therapy:

- **Combination Therapy:** Anti-angiogenic peptides are often used in combination with chemotherapy or radiation therapy to enhance treatment efficacy.

- **Metastasis Prevention:** By targeting tumor vasculature, anti-angiogenic peptides can help prevent metastasis by reducing the blood supply necessary for tumor growth in distant organs.

Examples of Anti-Angiogenic Peptides:

- **Endostatin:** Derived from the extracellular matrix protein collagen XVIII, endostatin inhibits endothelial cell proliferation and angiogenesis.

- **Angiostatin:** Fragment of plasminogen that blocks angiogenesis by inhibiting endothelial cell migration and inducing apoptosis.

- **Thrombospondin-1 Peptides:** Bind to CD36 receptors on endothelial cells, disrupting VEGF signaling and inhibiting angiogenesis.

Challenges and Future Directions

• **Delivery and Stability:** Enhancing peptide stability, bioavailability, and tissue penetration for effective tumor targeting.

• **Resistance Mechanisms:** Developing strategies to overcome resistance mechanisms that may develop against targeted peptides or anti-angiogenic therapies.

• **Clinical Translation:** Advancing preclinical findings into clinical trials to validate efficacy, safety, and therapeutic benefits in patients with different types and stages of cancer.

Tumor targeting and anti-angiogenic peptides represent promising avenues in cancer therapy, offering targeted approaches to inhibit tumor growth, metastasis, and angiogenesis while potentially minimizing side effects associated with traditional therapies. Continued research and clinical development are essential to harness the full therapeutic potential of these innovative peptide-based strategies in oncology.

Peptide Treatments For Heart Conditions

Peptides have shown promising applications in the treatment of various heart conditions, leveraging their ability to target specific mechanisms involved in cardiovascular diseases. Here's an overview of peptide treatments for heart conditions, focusing on their mechanisms of action and clinical applications:

Mechanisms of Action

Cardiac Remodeling and Function:

• Peptides can modulate cardiac remodeling processes, including hypertrophy and fibrosis, which are common in heart failure and other cardiac diseases.

• **Example:** Peptides targeting neurohormonal pathways (e.g., angiotensin II, endothelin-1) can inhibit pathological cardiac remodeling and improve cardiac function.

Vascular Function and Blood Pressure Regulation:

- Peptides may influence vascular tone and endothelial function, impacting blood pressure regulation and vascular health.

- **Example:** Peptides targeting endothelin receptors or nitric oxide pathways can enhance vasodilation and improve blood flow.

Ischemic Heart Disease and Angiogenesis:

- Peptides can promote angiogenesis and improve blood flow to ischemic heart tissues, supporting tissue repair and regeneration.

- **Example:** Peptides targeting vascular endothelial growth factor (VEGF) receptors can stimulate angiogenesis in ischemic myocardium.

Electrophysiological Stability:

- Peptides may modulate cardiac ion channels and electrical signaling, contributing to improved cardiac rhythm and reduced arrhythmias.

- **Example:** Peptides targeting potassium or calcium channels can stabilize cardiac electrophysiology and prevent arrhythmias.

Clinical Applications

Heart Failure:

- **Neurohormonal Modulation:** Peptides such as angiotensin-converting enzyme (ACE) inhibitors or angiotensin receptor blockers (ARBs) target the renin-angiotensin-aldosterone system (RAAS) to reduce cardiac workload and improve outcomes in heart failure patients.

- **Natriuretic Peptides:** Synthetic analogs of natriuretic peptides (e.g., atrial natriuretic peptide, B-type natriuretic peptide) are used to enhance diuresis and vasodilation, reducing fluid overload in heart failure.

Ischemic Heart Disease:

- **Angiogenic Peptides:** Peptides promoting angiogenesis (e.g., VEGF analogs) are investigated for enhancing collateral vessel formation and myocardial perfusion in ischemic heart disease.

- **Myocardial Protection:** Peptides targeting mitochondrial function or apoptosis pathways may protect myocardial tissue during ischemia-reperfusion injury.

Arrhythmias:

- **Ion Channel Modulators:** Peptides targeting ion channels (e.g., potassium channels) can stabilize cardiac electrophysiology and prevent arrhythmias in conditions like atrial fibrillation.

Challenges and Future Directions:

- **Peptide Stability and Delivery:** Improving peptide stability, bioavailability, and delivery methods to enhance efficacy and minimize degradation.

- **Clinical Validation:** Conducting rigorous clinical trials to establish safety, efficacy, and optimal dosing regimens for peptide-based therapies in different heart conditions.

- **Combination Therapies:** Exploring synergistic effects of peptides with conventional therapies (e.g., beta-blockers, statins) or other emerging treatments (e.g., gene therapy) for comprehensive management of heart diseases.

- **Personalized Medicine:** Developing personalized peptide therapies based on genetic profiles or biomarkers to tailor treatment strategies for individual patients.

Peptides offer diverse therapeutic strategies for managing heart conditions by targeting specific pathological mechanisms involved in cardiovascular diseases. Continued research and clinical advancements hold promise for expanding the role of peptide-based therapies in improving outcomes and quality of life for patients with heart conditions.

CHAPTER TEN
Vasodilators And Cardiac Peptides

Vasodilators and cardiac peptides play critical roles in cardiovascular physiology and pathology, influencing vascular tone, cardiac function, and overall cardiovascular health. Here's an exploration of vasodilators, cardiac peptides, and their interactions:

Vasodilators

- Vasodilators are substances that relax and widen blood vessels, thereby reducing blood pressure and improving blood flow. They play essential roles in regulating vascular tone and are used therapeutically to manage various cardiovascular conditions:

Mechanisms of Action:

• **Smooth Muscle Relaxation:** Vasodilators act directly on vascular smooth muscle cells to inhibit contraction and promote relaxation.

• **Endothelial Function:** Some vasodilators enhance nitric oxide (NO) release from endothelial cells, which relaxes vascular smooth muscle and dilates blood vessels.

• **Ion Channel Modulation:** Others act on ion channels (e.g., potassium channels) in vascular smooth muscle, leading to hyperpolarization and relaxation.

Types of Vasodilators:

- **Nitric Oxide (NO) Donors:** Drugs that release NO or mimic its effects, such as nitroglycerin and sodium nitroprusside.

- **Calcium Channel Blockers:** Agents that inhibit calcium influx into smooth muscle cells, leading to relaxation, e.g., verapamil and diltiazem.

- **Potassium Channel Openers:** Drugs that open potassium channels, hyperpolarizing smooth muscle cells, e.g., minoxidil.

Clinical Applications:

- **Hypertension:** Vasodilators are used to reduce blood pressure in hypertensive patients, improving cardiovascular outcomes and reducing risk of complications.

- **Heart Failure:** They can alleviate symptoms by reducing cardiac workload and improving cardiac output.

- **Angina Pectoris:** Vasodilators like nitroglycerin relieve anginal symptoms by increasing coronary blood flow and reducing myocardial oxygen demand.

Cardiac Peptides:

• Cardiac peptides are hormones or signaling molecules primarily produced by the heart, influencing cardiovascular function through various physiological mechanisms:

Types of Cardiac Peptides:

Atrial Natriuretic Peptide (ANP) and B-type Natriuretic Peptide (BNP):

- **Role:** Released in response to atrial or ventricular stretch due to increased blood volume or pressure.

- **Mechanism:** ANP and BNP promote natriuresis (sodium excretion), diuresis (water excretion), and vasodilation to reduce blood volume and pressure.

C-Type Natriuretic Peptide (CNP):

- **Role:** Expressed primarily in endothelial cells and involved in vascular homeostasis and relaxation.

- **Mechanism:** CNP acts as a vasodilator and regulator of vascular tone, influencing blood flow and endothelial function.

Clinical Applications:

- **Heart Failure:** Measurement of BNP or NT-proBNP levels aids in diagnosis, prognosis, and management of heart failure.

- **Hypertension:** Some peptides like ANP and CNP have vasodilatory effects, contributing to blood pressure regulation.

- **Cardioprotection:** Peptides may exert cardioprotective effects by reducing cardiac hypertrophy, fibrosis, and remodeling.

Interactions and Synergies

- **Synergistic Effects:** Vasodilators and cardiac peptides often exhibit complementary actions in regulating vascular tone and cardiac function.

- **Example:** ANP and BNP can augment the vasodilatory effects of exogenous NO donors or enhance the responsiveness of vascular smooth muscle to calcium channel blockers.

Therapeutic Strategies:

- **Combination Therapies:** Using vasodilators alongside therapies that modulate cardiac peptides (e.g., ACE inhibitors or angiotensin receptor blockers that increase BNP levels) for comprehensive management of hypertension or heart failure.

- **Targeted Approaches:** Developing novel therapies that combine vasodilator properties with peptides that target specific cardiac receptors or signaling pathways involved in cardiovascular diseases.

Challenges and Future Directions:

• **Optimizing Therapy:** Identifying the optimal balance and combination of vasodilators and cardiac peptides for personalized treatment based on patient-specific cardiovascular profiles.

• **Drug Delivery:** Enhancing delivery methods to maximize the bioavailability and efficacy of peptides in targeted cardiovascular therapies.

• **Clinical Validation:** Conducting rigorous clinical trials to validate the safety, efficacy, and long-term benefits of combined vasodilator and peptide-based therapies in cardiovascular diseases.

Vasodilators and cardiac peptides represent pivotal components in the management of cardiovascular diseases, offering diverse therapeutic strategies to regulate vascular tone, improve cardiac function, and enhance patient outcomes. Continued research and innovation are essential to unlock the full therapeutic potential of these approaches in cardiovascular medicine.

Peptides In Dermatology And Wound Care

Peptides have gained significant attention in dermatology and wound care due to their diverse biological activities and potential therapeutic applications in skin health, wound healing, and cosmetic dermatology. Here's an overview of how peptides are utilized in these fields:

Dermatology

Anti-Aging and Skin Repair:

- **Collagen Synthesis:** Peptides like palmitoyl pentapeptide-4 (Matrixyl) stimulate collagen synthesis, promoting skin firmness and reducing wrinkles.

- **Elastin Production:** Certain peptides enhance elastin production, improving skin elasticity and reducing sagging.

- **Barrier Function:** Peptides can strengthen the skin barrier by promoting lipid synthesis and enhancing barrier repair mechanisms.

Anti-Inflammatory and Antioxidant Properties:

- Peptides such as thymosin beta-4 and copper peptides exhibit anti-inflammatory effects, reducing redness and inflammation associated with skin conditions like rosacea or eczema.

- Antioxidant peptides scavenge free radicals, protecting skin cells from oxidative stress and premature aging.

Pigmentation Control:

- Peptides like oligopeptide-68 or acetyl hexapeptide-8 (Argireline) inhibit melanin synthesis, helping to lighten hyperpigmentation and age spots.

Cosmetic Applications:

- Peptides are common ingredients in cosmetic formulations for moisturizing, skin rejuvenation, and improving overall skin texture and appearance.

Wound Care

Wound Healing:

- **Collagen Stimulation:** Peptides that mimic collagen fragments (e.g., KTTKS) promote fibroblast migration and collagen synthesis, accelerating wound closure.

- **Angiogenesis:** Certain peptides stimulate angiogenesis (formation of new blood vessels), improving blood flow to the wound area and enhancing tissue repair.

- **Antimicrobial Activity:** Some peptides have antimicrobial properties, helping to prevent infection in wounds.

Scar Reduction:

- Peptides like copper tripeptide-1 (GHK-Cu) modulate inflammation and promote remodeling of extracellular matrix, reducing scar formation and improving cosmetic outcomes post-wound healing.

Chronic Wounds and Ulcers:

- Peptide-based dressings or topical formulations are explored for treating chronic wounds like diabetic ulcers or venous ulcers, enhancing healing rates and reducing complications.

Advances and Challenges

Peptide Design and Delivery:

- Designing peptides with optimal sequences and structures to enhance stability, bioavailability, and skin penetration remains a challenge.

- Delivery systems such as nanotechnology or liposomal formulations are explored to improve peptide delivery to target tissues effectively.

Clinical Validation:

- Conducting robust clinical trials to demonstrate the efficacy and safety of peptide-based therapies in dermatological conditions and wound care settings.

- Establishing standardized protocols for peptide treatment regimens and formulations tailored to specific patient needs.

Regulatory Considerations:

- Meeting regulatory requirements for peptide-based products in dermatology and wound care, including safety profiles, manufacturing standards, and labeling requirements.

Personalized Medicine:

• Developing personalized peptide therapies based on individual skin types, wound characteristics, and patient responses to optimize treatment outcomes.

Peptides offer promising therapeutic avenues in dermatology and wound care, leveraging their biological activities to enhance skin health, promote wound healing, and address various dermatological conditions. Continued research and innovation are crucial to unlock the full potential of peptides in these fields and translate discoveries into effective clinical applications.

CHAPTER ELEVEN
Cosmeceuticals And Regenerative Medicine

Cosmeceuticals and regenerative medicine represent two intertwined fields aimed at enhancing skin health, appearance, and regeneration through advanced scientific approaches. Here's an overview of how these areas intersect and their applications:

Cosmeceuticals

Definition and Purpose:

- **Cosmeceuticals** are cosmetic products containing biologically active ingredients that offer therapeutic benefits beyond traditional skincare.

- They bridge the gap between cosmetics and pharmaceuticals, offering ingredients like peptides, antioxidants, vitamins, and botanical extracts that provide anti-aging, moisturizing, and protective effects.

Key Ingredients in Cosmeceuticals:

- **Peptides:** Peptides such as Matrixyl (palmitoyl pentapeptide-4) stimulate collagen synthesis, reducing wrinkles and improving skin elasticity.

• **Antioxidants:** Vitamins C and E, coenzyme Q10, and green tea extracts neutralize free radicals, preventing oxidative damage and premature aging.

• **Retinoids:** Vitamin A derivatives like retinol promote cell turnover, improving skin texture and reducing fine lines.

• **Botanical Extracts:** Plant-derived compounds (e.g., green tea, licorice root) with anti-inflammatory, soothing, and brightening properties.

Benefits:

• **Anti-Aging:** Cosmeceuticals target signs of aging such as wrinkles, fine lines, and loss of firmness by promoting collagen synthesis and improving skin hydration.

- **Skin Repair:** Active ingredients support skin barrier function, enhance moisture retention, and accelerate cell turnover for smoother, healthier skin.

- **Skin Protection:** Antioxidants and UV filters protect against environmental stressors like UV radiation and pollution, reducing photoaging and skin damage.

Clinical Evidence and Validation:

- Cosmeceutical formulations are often supported by clinical studies demonstrating their efficacy in improving skin appearance and health.

- Long-term use may show benefits in reducing signs of aging and maintaining skin integrity, depending on formulation and individual skin type.

<u>Regenerative Medicine</u>

Definition and Principles:

- **Regenerative Medicine** focuses on repairing or replacing damaged tissues and organs using biological approaches, including stem cells, growth factors, and tissue engineering.

- It aims to restore normal function and structure to tissues affected by injury, disease, or aging.

Applications in Dermatology:

- **Stem Cell Therapy:** Stem cells derived from adipose tissue or bone marrow are used to regenerate skin cells, improve wound healing, and stimulate collagen production.

- **Platelet-Rich Plasma (PRP):** PRP contains growth factors that promote tissue repair and collagen synthesis, used in facial rejuvenation and hair restoration.

- **Exosome Therapy:** Exosomes derived from stem cells deliver bioactive molecules (proteins, RNAs) to target cells, enhancing skin regeneration and anti-aging effects.

Emerging Technologies:

- **3D Bioprinting:** Enables precise fabrication of skin substitutes or tissue constructs for wound healing and cosmetic purposes.

- **Gene Editing:** CRISPR technology may allow targeted modifications of skin cells to correct genetic defects or enhance therapeutic properties in regenerative medicine.

Challenges and Future Directions:

• **Safety and Efficacy:** Ensuring the safety and efficacy of regenerative treatments in cosmetic and medical settings through rigorous preclinical and clinical studies.

• **Standardization:** Developing standardized protocols for regenerative therapies to optimize outcomes and minimize variability.

• **Ethical Considerations:** Addressing ethical concerns related to stem cell use, genetic manipulation, and long-term effects of regenerative treatments.

<u>Integration and Synergies:</u>

- **Combined Approaches:** Integrating cosmeceutical ingredients with regenerative therapies (e.g., peptides with stem cell-derived growth factors) may enhance treatment outcomes by synergistically promoting skin regeneration, anti-aging effects, and overall skin health.

- **Personalized Treatments:** Tailoring cosmeceutical and regenerative therapies based on individual skin characteristics, genetic factors, and specific skin concerns to optimize efficacy and patient satisfaction.

Cosmeceuticals and regenerative medicine represent innovative approaches in dermatology aimed at improving skin health, appearance, and regenerative capabilities through advanced scientific and biotechnological advancements. Continued research and development in these fields hold promise for transforming skincare and rejuvenation therapies, offering personalized solutions for diverse cosmetic and therapeutic needs.

Issues In Peptide Stability And Bioavailability

Peptides, despite their therapeutic potential, face significant challenges related to stability and bioavailability, which are crucial for their effectiveness in clinical applications. Here are some key issues and considerations in peptide stability and bioavailability:

Issues in Peptide Stability

Proteolytic Degradation:

- Peptides are susceptible to enzymatic degradation by proteases present in biological fluids (e.g., plasma, gastrointestinal tract).

- **Solution:** Designing peptides with D-amino acids or modified amino acids can enhance resistance to enzymatic degradation.

Chemical Instability:

- Peptides may undergo chemical degradation due to oxidation, hydrolysis, or deamidation, affecting their structural integrity and biological activity.

- **Solution:** Formulating peptides with stabilizing agents (e.g., antioxidants, chelating agents) or modifying peptide sequences to enhance stability against chemical degradation.

Aggregation and Denaturation:

- Peptides can aggregate or denature under certain conditions (e.g., temperature, pH extremes), leading to loss of bioactivity.

- **Solution:** Optimizing formulation conditions (e.g., pH, buffer composition) and storage conditions (e.g., temperature, freeze-drying) to prevent aggregation and maintain peptide stability.

- **Poor Solubility:** Some peptides exhibit poor solubility in aqueous solutions, limiting their bioavailability and practical use in formulations.

- **Solution:** Modifying peptide sequences to enhance solubility or using solubilizing agents (e.g., surfactants, co-solvents) in formulation development.

Issues in Peptide Bioavailability

Absorption Barriers:

• Peptides administered orally face challenges in crossing the gastrointestinal epithelium due to enzymatic degradation and poor membrane permeability.

• **Solution:** Developing peptide analogs or prodrugs that enhance oral absorption or using alternative routes (e.g., subcutaneous, intravenous) for systemic delivery.

Distribution and Clearance:

• Peptides may exhibit rapid distribution and clearance from circulation, limiting their duration of action and therapeutic efficacy.

• **Solution:** Formulating peptides with longer half-lives (e.g., pegylation, lipidation) or developing sustained-release formulations to prolong systemic exposure.

Immunogenicity and Tolerance:

- Peptides can induce immune responses or tolerance, affecting their safety and efficacy upon repeated administration.

- **Solution:** Designing peptides with reduced immunogenic potential (e.g., modifying sequences, incorporating non-immunogenic epitopes) or using immunomodulatory agents to enhance tolerance.

Strategies to Improve Peptide Stability and Bioavailability

Peptide Modification:

• Structural modifications (e.g., cyclization, amidation) can enhance stability and biological activity.

• Using unnatural amino acids or peptidomimetics to improve proteolytic resistance and pharmacokinetic properties.

Delivery Systems:

• Utilizing delivery systems such as nanoparticles, liposomes, or micelles to protect peptides from enzymatic degradation and facilitate targeted delivery to specific tissues.

Chemical Modification:

- Conjugating peptides with polymers (e.g., polyethylene glycol, PEGylation) or lipid moieties to improve solubility, stability, and bioavailability.

Formulation Optimization:

- Fine-tuning formulation parameters (e.g., pH, buffer composition, excipients) to optimize peptide stability, solubility, and delivery characteristics.

Biophysical Characterization:

- Employing biophysical techniques (e.g., mass spectrometry, nuclear magnetic resonance) to study peptide structure, stability, and interactions with biological targets.

Future Directions:

- **Advanced Drug Delivery Systems:** Developing innovative delivery systems that enhance peptide stability, bioavailability, and tissue targeting.

- **Bioinformatics and Rational Design:** Utilizing computational tools to predict peptide stability, optimize sequences, and design novel analogs with improved pharmacokinetic profiles.

- **Clinical Translation:** Conducting rigorous preclinical and clinical studies to validate the safety, efficacy, and therapeutic potential of peptide-based therapies in diverse disease indications.

It is imperative to resolve concerns regarding peptide bioavailability and stability in order to optimize their therapeutic potential in clinical applications. The full therapeutic benefits of peptides in medicine and biotechnology are contingent upon the successful resolution of these challenges through advancements in peptide design, formulation technologies, and delivery systems.

Disclaimer:

The information contained in this book is for educational and informational purposes only and is not intended as medical advice. Peptide therapy is a complex and evolving field, and the content provided herein is based on current research and knowledge as of the publication date. Readers are encouraged to consult with a qualified healthcare professional before starting any new therapy or treatment.

The authors and publishers of this book are not responsible for any adverse effects or consequences resulting from the use of the information presented. The content should not be used as a substitute for professional medical advice, diagnosis, or treatment. The reader should always seek the guidance of a licensed healthcare provider with any questions regarding a medical condition or treatment options.

Furthermore, the efficacy and safety of peptide therapies can vary based on individual health conditions and circumstances. The regulatory status of peptide treatments may also differ by country and region. It is the reader's responsibility to ensure compliance with local laws and regulations regarding the use of peptide therapies.

By reading this book, you acknowledge and agree that the authors, publishers, and any affiliates are not liable for any claim or loss, direct or indirect, arising from the use or misuse of the information provided.

Note: Always consult a healthcare professional for medical advice and treatment tailored to your specific needs.

Conclusion

Peptides exhibit significant potential as therapeutic agents in a variety of disciplines, such as dermatology, wound care, regenerative medicine, and beyond.

They are valuable candidates for addressing complex medical challenges and improving patient outcomes due to their distinctive properties, including biocompatibility, specificity, and diverse biological activities. Nevertheless, the widespread adoption of peptide-based therapies is impeded by substantial obstacles, particularly those associated with bioavailability and stability.

The efficacy and practical application of peptides are restricted by their susceptibility to enzymatic degradation, chemical instability, and inadequate absorption. Innovative approaches to peptide design, formulation, and delivery systems are necessary to surmount these obstacles.

The incorporation of stabilizing agents, modification of amino acid sequences, and the development of sophisticated delivery technologies are among the recent advancements in peptide engineering that offer optimistic solutions to improve bioavailability and enhance peptide stability.

Furthermore, our comprehension of peptide behavior is being amplified by ongoing research in biophysics, pharmacokinetics, and computational modeling, which is enabling the creation of customized therapies. In order to realize the complete therapeutic potential of peptides, it is imperative to maintain an ongoing investment in research and development.

Peptides can facilitate personalized medicine, targeted therapies, and innovative treatments that address unmet medical requirements across diverse disease areas by surmounting stability and bioavailability obstacles. In conclusion, peptides are on the brink of revolutionizing healthcare with their precise, potent, and versatile therapeutic applications, despite the obstacles they must surmount.

Dr. Kyren Steven's Approach:

Dr. Kyren Steven's approach to peptides therapy is rooted in personalized medicine. He carefully evaluates each patient's unique health profile and tailors peptide treatments to meet their specific needs. His protocols often involve a combination of peptides to achieve synergistic effects and optimize therapeutic outcomes.

Safety and Efficacy:

Safety and efficacy are paramount in Dr. Steven's practice. He emphasizes the importance of using high-quality, clinically tested peptides and monitors patients closely to ensure optimal results and minimize potential side effects. His research and clinical experience contribute to the growing body of evidence supporting the benefits of peptides therapy.

THE END

www.ingramcontent.com/pod-product-compliance
Lightning Source LLC
Chambersburg PA
CBHW071829210526
45479CB00001B/57